Differential Diagnosis in General Medicine

Differential Diagnosis in General Medicine

Ahran Arnold

The University of Buckingham Press

First published in Great Britain in 2013 by

The University of Buckingham Press
Yeomanry House
Hunter Street
Buckingham MK18 1EG

© Ahran Arnold

The moral right of the author has been asserted.

All rights reserved. No part of this publication may be reproduced, stored or introduced into a retrieval system or transmitted in any form or by any means without the prior permission of the publisher nor may be circulated in any form of binding or cover other than the one in which it is published and without a similar condition including this condition being imposed on the subsequent purchaser.

A CIP catalogue record for this book is available at the British Library

ISBN 978-1-908684-39-4

Printed and bound in Great Britain by Marston Book Services Ltd, Oxfordshire

Introduction

Appreciation of the differential diagnosis for a particular symptom or sign has been a pillar of the practice of general medicine for generations of doctors. This has never been more true than now, in the modern NHS with its focus on patient safety.

Keeping a broad differential in mind when approaching the new patient is often key to avoid pitfalls of tunnel vision in management. Equally, the importance of the differential diagnosis in undergraduate and postgraduate examinations cannot be understated.

This book contains a series of lists of differential diagnoses for general medical presentations. We hope it will be of use for doctors wishing to refresh their memory with a quick reference guide, students of undergraduate medicine as well as postgraduate doctors in preparation for Membership of the Royal College of Physicians (MRCP) examinations.

The best way to navigate the book is to identify the symptom or clinical feature required using the contents pages but the lists can be read in sequence for the general reader.

A Arnold

Contents

Abdominal mass	1
Abdominal pain	2
Abnormal gait	4
Absent radial pulse	5
Alopecia	6
Acute Renal Failure	7
Ascites	9
Atypical pneumonia	11
Autonomic neuropathy	12
B12 deficiency	13
Back pain	14
Bacterial meningitis: causative bacteria	15
Bilateral hilar lymphadenopathy	16
Bleeding disorder	17
Bradycardia	18
Cardiac Syncope	19
Cardiac valve vegetations	20
Carpal tunnel syndrome	21
Cerebellar syndrome	22
Charcot's joints	23
Chest Pain	24
Coma	26
Congenital heart disease	28
Constipation	29
Cord Compression	30
Cough	31
Crackles	32
Chronic Renal Failure	33
Chromosomal abnormalities with cardiac abnormalities	35

Contents

Diarrhoea	36
Dysarthria	39
Dysphagia	40
Dyspnoea	42
Eosinophilia	44
Erythema nodosum	45
Facial paralysis	46
Finger Clubbing	47
Generalised Lymphadenopathy	49
Glomerulonephritis	50
Glomerulonephritis	51
Haematuria	52
Haemolytic anaemia	53
Haemoptysis	54
Headache (Chronic)	55
Headache (acute onset)	56
Complete (3rd degree) Heart Block	57
Hepatic encephalopathy –precipitants	58
Hepatomegaly	59
Horner's Syndrome	62
Hyperpigmentation	63
Hypertension	64
Hyperviscosity syndrome	66
Hypoglycaemia	67
Hypothyroidism	68
Intestinal obstruction	69
JVP elevation	70
Knee pain	71
Koilonychia	72
Lactic acidosis	73
Leg ulcers	74
Liver Cirrhosis	75

Contents

Left Ventricular Failure	76
Macrocytic anaemia	78
Malabsorbtion	79
Mouth ulcers (Apthous)	81
Muscular dystrophies	82
Myopathy	83
Nephrotic syndrome	84
Neurocutaneous syndromes	85
Neutrophilia	86
Normocytic anaemia	87
Nystagmaus	88
Obstructive Jaundice	89
Optic atrophy	90
Pancytopenia	91
Papilloedema	92
Pericarditis	93
Peripheral Neuropathy	95
Peroneal Nerve palsy	97
Pleural effusion	98
Polycythaemia	99
Polyuria	100
Proteinuria	101
Proximal myopathy	102
Purpura	103
Pyrexia of unknown origin	104
Acute Coronary Syndrome	106
Splenomegaly	107
Seronegative arthritis	109
Seronegative arthritis	110
Spastic paraparesis	111
Seronegative Arthritides	112
Syncope	113

Contents

Tachycardia- Broad complex	115
Tachycardia- Narrow complex	116
Testicular pain	117
Thrombocytosis	118
Thrombophilia	119
Tremor	120
Uveitis	121
Vasculitis	122
Vomiting	123
Wide splitting of heart sounds	125

Differential Diagnosis in General Medicine

Abdominal mass

Left

Transplanted kidney

Diverticular abscess

Carcinoma Colon

Right

Crohn's disease

Appendular abscess

Ovarian tumour

Caecal cancer

Lymph nodes

Abdominal pain

- Appendicitis
- Gastritis
- Peptic ulcer disease
- Cholecystitis
- Pancreatitis
- Renal colic
- Abdominal Aortic Aneurysm
- Obstruction of small or large intestine
- Hepatitis
- Pyelonephritis

Differential Diagnosis in General Medicine

Abdominal pain (continued)

Diverticulitis

Salpingitis

Cystitis

Ruptured ectopic pregnancy

Malignancy

Inflammatory Bowel Disease

Irritable Bowel Syndrome

Peritonitis

Abnormal gait

Upper motor neuron hemiplegia

Parkinson's disease (shuffling gait)

Cerebellar lesions (broad based gait)

Spastic paraplegia

Posterior column lesion
(positive Romberg's test)
B12 deficiency
Syphillis

High stepping gait (foot drop)

Proximal Myopathy (waddling gait)

Involuntary movements
Chorea
Athetosis
Dystonia
Hemiballismus

Differential Diagnosis in General Medicine

Absent radial pulse

- Subclavian artery stenosis
- Blalock-taussig shunt
- Takayasu's arteritis
- Embolism
- Aberrant vessels
- Catheterization of brachial artery

Alopecia

- Drugs
- Telogen effluvium
- Alopecia areata
- Iron deficiency
- Hypothyoidism

Acute Renal Failure

Pre renal

Hypovolaemia

Renal Artery Stenosis

Renal

Acute tubular necrosis

Vasculitis

Accelerated hypertension

Haemolytic uraemic syndrome

Thrombotic thrombocytopenic purpura

Pre-eclampsia

Acute Renal Failure (continued)

Glomerulonephritis

Drugs

Pyelonephritis

Gout

Post renal

Obstructive uropathy

Ascites

Liver cirrhosis

Malignancy

Hypoalbuminaemia
(eg. nephrotic syndrome)

Tuberculosis

Congestive Cardiac Failure

Constrictive pericarditis

Chylous Ascites
(obstructed lymph flow)

Pancreatic ascites
(acute pancreatitis)

Budd-Chiari syndrome
(thrombosis of hepatic vein)

Ascites (continued)

Ruptured ectopic pregnancy

Meig's syndrome
(ovarian tumour)

Atypical pneumonia

Mycoplasma

Legionella

Viral
(Cytomegalovirus, Coxsackie, Echo. Varicella)

Chlamydia

Autonomic neuropathy

- Diabetes mellitus
- Shy Drager Syndrome
- Parkinson's Disease
- Guillain – Barre Syndrome
- Tabes Dorsalis
- Familial Dysautonomia

B12 deficiency

Pernicious anaemia

Vegetarians

Ileal resection
(post gastrectomy)

Crohn's disease

Coeliac disease

Tape worm
(Diphyllobothrium latum)

Back pain

Disc prolapse

Trauma

Facet joint syndrome

Ankylosing spondylitis

Spinal fracture

Tumour
(primary, secondary)

Mechanical (postural)

Bacterial meningitis: causative bacteria

Haemophilus influenza

Streptococcus pneumonia

Neisseria Meningitidis

Listeria monocytogenes

Bilateral hilar lymphadenopathy

- Sarcoidosis
- Tuberculosis
- Lymphoma
- Carcinoma

Bleeding disorder

Haemophilia

Idiopathic Thrombocytopaenic Purpura

Aplastic anaemia

Vitamin K deficiency – Liver disease

Vascular
(Osler-Rendu-Weber, Ehlers Danlos)

Von Willebrand's Disease

Senile purpura

Henoch schonlein purpura

Thrombotic thrombocytopenic purpura

Bradycardia

Drugs

Hypothyroidism

Increased intra-cranial pressure

Hypothermia

Hyperkalaemia

Complete heart block

Cardiac Syncope

Vasovagal syncope

Postural hypotension

Micturition syncope

Carotid sinus syncope

Aortic stenosis

Hypertrophic Obstructive Cardiomyopathy

Fallot's tetralogy

Tachycardia

Stokes-adams attack (bradycardia)

Sinus pauses

Pacemaker failure

Cardiac valve vegetations

Infective Endocarditis

Libman Sachs Endocarditis
(Systemic Lupus Erythematosus)

Marantic endocarditis

Valve myxoma

Ruptured chordae tendinae

Carpal tunnel syndrome

- Hypothyroidism
- Rheumatoid arthritis
- Diabetes Mellitus
- Acromegaly
- Obesity

Cerebellar syndrome

- Alcohol
- Multiple sclerosis
- Arnold-Chiari malformation
- Friedreich's ataxia
- Cerebellar tumour
- Acoustic neuroma
- Cerebellar Stroke
- Basilar invagination
- Anti-epileptic drugs
- Hypothyroidism

Charcot's joints

- Diabetic neuropathy
- Tabes dorsalis
- Syringomyelia
- Hereditary sensory neuropathy
- Leprosy

Chest Pain

- Acute Coronary Syndrome
- Angina
- Pericarditis
- Pulmonary Embolism
- Gastro-Oesophageal Reflux Disease
- Oesophageal spasm
- Pneumothorax
- Aortic Dissection
- Pneumonia
- Myocarditis

Differential Diagnosis in General Medicine

> **Chest Pain (continued)**

> Tietze's Syndrome (costochondritis)
>
> Herpes Zoster
>
> Trauma
>
> Mediastinitis

Coma

- Head Trauma
- Epilepsy
- Drug Overdose
- Alcohol
- Cerebrovascular Accident
- Hypoglycaemia
- Meningitis
- Encephalitis
- Hepatic coma
- Septicaemia

Coma (continued)

Renal Failure

Hypothyroidism

Electrolyte imbalance

Hypo/hyper thermia

Diabetic Ketoacidosis

Hyperosmolar non-ketotic coma

Adrenal Failure

Raised intracranial pressure

Congenital heart disease

Ventricular Septal Defect

Atrial Septal Defect

Patent Ductus Arteriosus

Pulmonary stenosis

Coarctation of aorta

Aortic stenosis

Fallot's tetralogy

Transposition of great vessels

(many other abnormalities)

Differential Diagnosis in General Medicine

Constipation

- Hypothyroidism
- Hypercalcaemia
- Idiopathic slow transit
- Irritable Bowel Syndrome
- Drugs
- Parkinson's disease
- Cord compression
- Hirschprung's Disease
- Megarectum

Cord Compression

- Metastatic malignancy
- Tuberculosis
- Disc prolapse
- Abscess (extradural)
- Glioma
- Neurofibroma

Cough

- Tuberculosis
- Pneumonia
- Chronic Obrtructive Pulmonary DIsease
- Acute bronchitis
- Bornchiectasis
- Bronchial Carcinoma
- Aspergillosis
- Variant Asthma

Crackles

- Left Ventricular Failure
- Fibrosing alveolitis
- Extrinsic allergic alveolitis
- Pneumonia
- Bronchiectasis

Chronic Renal Failure

Diabetic nephropathy

Hypertension

Reno-vascular disease

Vasculitis

Pyelonephritis

Post glomerulonephritis

Polycystic kidney disease

Multiple myeloma

Chronic Renal Failure (continued)

Urinary tract obstruction
eg benign prostatic hyperplasia
Prostatic carcinoma

Retroperitoneal fibrosis

Sickle cell anaemia

Drugs

Analgesic nephropathy

Chromosomal abnormalities with cardiac abnormalities

Down's Syndrome
(Trisomy 21)– Atrial Septal Defect, Ventricular Septal Defect, Fallot's tetralogy

Turner's syndrome
(XO) – Coarctation of aorta, bicuspid valve

Diarrhoea

Gastroenteritis
(Viral, Campylobacter jejuni/salmonella E.coli)

Inflammatory Bowel Disease

Pseudomembraneous Colitis

Diverticulitis

Ischaemic colitis

Drugs

Irritable Bowel Syndrome

Diarrhoea (continued)

Endocrine
Carcinoid
VIPoma
Thyrotoxicosis

Diabetic Autonomic neuropathy

Purgative abuse

Colonic carcinoma

Tropical diarrhoea
Amoebiasis
Cholera
Giardia

Shigellosis

Behcet's disease

Diarrhoea (continued)

- Intestinal lymhoma
- Bile acid malabsorption
- Medullary carcinoma of thyroid

Dysarthria

- Bulbar palsy
- Pseudobulbar palsy
- Cerebellar lesions
- Facial muscle paralysis or weakness
- Basal ganglia lesion
- Loose dentures

Dysphagia

- Carcinoma of the oesophagus
- Benign stricture
- Foreign body
- Pharyngeal pouch
- Pharyngeal web
- Scleroderma
- Myasthenia Gravis
- Parkinson's disease
- Bulbar Palsy

Dysphagia (continued)

Pseudobulbar palsy

Extrinsic compression
(eg. Thymoma, retrosternal goitre,
bronchial carcinoma, aortic aneurysm,
lymph nodes, enlarged left atrium)

Achalasia

Dysmotility due to Diabetes or
Chagas' disease

Dyspnoea

Left heart failure

Chronic Obstructive Pulmonary Disease

Asthma

Pneumonia

Tuberculosis

Aspergillosis

Extrinsic allergic alveolitis

Fibrosing Alveolitis

Lung Collapse

Dyspnoea (continued)

Pneumothorax

Pleural effusion

Foreign body

Eosinophilia

Drugs

Asthma

Helminth infection

Skin diseases eg psoriasis

Lymphoma

Loffler's syndrome

Erythema nodosum

- Streptococcal infection
- Tuberculosis
- Sarcoidosis
- Drugs
- Penicillin
- Inflammatory bowel disease
- Leptospirosis
- Yersinia
- Leprosy

Facial paralysis

Stroke

Nuclear tumour or vasculitis

Bell's palsy

Parotid tumour

Acoustic neuroma

Trauma

Meningioma

Differential Diagnosis in General Medicine

Finger Clubbing

Cardiac
- Congenital Cyanotic Heart Disease
- Infective Endocarditis
- Atrial Myxoma

Respiratory
- Bronchiectasis
- Fibrosing Alveolitis
- Bronchial Carcinoma
- Lung Abscess,/Empyema
- Pulmonary fibrosis
- Pulmonary Hypertension

Gastrointestinal
- Inflammatory Bowel Disease
- Crohn's Disease
- Liver cirrhosis
- Coeliac Disease

Finger Clubbing (continued)

Endocrine
 Hyperthroidism (thyroid acropachy)

+ Hypertrophic Pulmonary Osteo-Arthritis

Generalised Lymphadenopathy

Lymphoma

Leukaemia

Metastatic malignancy

Infections: Glandular fever (Infectious Mononucleosis), TB, Syphillis, Toxoplasmosis, Viral infections

Sarcoidosis

Connective Tissue Disease eg Rheumatoid Arthritis, Systemic Lupus Erythematosus (SLE)

Chronic Skin sepsis

Glomerulonephritis

IgA Nephropathy

Henoch Schonlein Purpura

Proliferative Glomerulonephritis – focal, diffuse, mesangio capillary

SLE

Rapidly progressive Glomerulonephritis

Anti-Glomerular Basement Membrane disease

Glomerulonephritis

Physiological (puberty, pregnancy)

Autoimmune
Grave's disease
Hashimoto's disease

Thyroiditis

Acute de Quervain's Thyroiditis

Iodine deficiency

Multinodular goiter

Solitary nodular

Tumour

Tuberculosis

Haematuria

- Urinary tract infection
- Glomerulonephritis
- Drugs
- Polycystic Kidneys
- Calculi
- Bladder carcinoma
- Renal cell carcinoma

Haemolytic anaemia

Autoimmune – warm, cold

Paroxysmal cold haemoglobinuria

G6PD deficiency

Lymphoma

Hereditary spherocytosis

sickle cell anaemia

Thalassaemia

Malaria

Drugs

Haemoptysis

- Bronchial carcinoma
- Tuberculosis
- Bronchiectasis
- Pulmonary embolism
- Mitral stenosis
- Anticoagulants
- Bronchial adenoma
- Idiopathic pulmonary haemosiderosis

Headache (Chronic)

Migraine

Cluster headaches

Sinusitis

Giant cell arteritis

Brain tumour

Subdural haematoma

TB meningitis

Trigeminal neuralgia

Carbon monoxide poisoning

Hypertension
(Phaeochromocytoma)

Headache (acute onset)

Subarachnoid haemorrhage

Meningitis

Giant cell arteritis

Acute haemorrhagic stroke
Hypertensive encephalopathy

Migraine

Complete (3rd degree) Heart Block

- Ischaemia
- Myocardial Infarction
- Drugs
- Aortic Stenosis
- Infective Endocarditis
- Chaga's disease (Trypanosomiasis)

Hepatic encephalopathy – precipitants

Protein load – acute bleed

Electrolyte abnormalities

Drugs

Sepsis

Onset of Hepatocellular carcinoma

Hepatomegaly

Cirrhosis (early stages)

Infection
- Viral hepatitis
- Weil's disease (leptospirosis)
- Amoebiasis
- Hydatid cyst
- Multiple bacterial liver abscesses

Malignancy
- Metastases
- Hepatocellular carcinoma
- Cholangiocarcinoma
- Lymphoma

Hepatomegaly (continued)

Haematological
- Leukaemia
- Myelofibrosis
- Lymphoma
- Thalassaemia

Alcoholic liver disease

Fatty liver

Liver congestion
- Congestive cardiac failure
- Budd-Chiari syndrome (thrombosis of the hepatic vein)

Infilitrative disorder
- Sarcoidosis
- Amyloidosis

Differential Diagnosis in General Medicine

Hepatomegaly (continued)

Bile duct obstruction

Carcinoma of the head of the pancreas

Horner's Syndrome

Bronchial Carcinoma

Cervical sympathectomy

Aortic Aneurysm

Syringomyelia

Brachial Plexus Injury

Hyperpigmentation

Addison's

Haemochromatosis

Uraemia

Drugs

Ochronosis

Hypertension

Essential

Secondary

Endocrine
- Phaeochromocytoma
- Cushing's Syndrome
- Conn's Syndrome
- Acromegaly
- Congenital adrenal hyperplasia
- hyperparathyroidism

Renal Disease
- Renal Artery Stenosis
- Diabetic Nephropathy
- Adult Polycystic Kidney disease

Hypertension (continued)

Pregnancy
- Pre-eclampsia

Drugs
- Non-steroidal anti-inflammatories
- Oral contraceptive pill
- Steroids

Others
- Coarctation of Aorta
- Increased intra-cranial pressure
- Primary Polycythaemia

Hyperviscosity syndrome

Polycythaemia

Leukaemia

Waldenstrom's

Myeloma

Hypoglycaemia

Drugs – sulphonylurea

Alcohol

Hypopituitarism

Insulinoma

Addison's disease

Acute Liver failure

Hypothyroidism

Primary atrophic

Hashimoto's thyroiditis

Iodine deficiency

Drugs

Secondary hypothyroidism from hypopituitarism

Differential Diagnosis in General Medicine

Intestinal obstruction

Small intestine
- Adhesions
- Hernia
- Crohn's disease
- Intussuception
- Carcinoma

Large intestine
- Carcinoma
- Sigmoid voluvulus
- Diverticular disease

JVP elevation

- Congestive cardiac failure
- Tricuspid regurgitation
- Cor Pulmonale
- Superior Vena Cava obstruction

Knee pain

Ligament injury

Miniscal tear

Osteoarthritis

Rheumatoid arthritis

Gout

Ruptured baker's cyst

Septic arthritis

Referred hip pain

Reiter's syndrome

Koilonychia

Iron deficiency

Fungal nail infection

Raynaud's

Lactic acidosis

Shock with hypoperfusion

Severe hypoxia

Hepatic/renal failure

Drugs
(metformin)

Diabetes Mellitus

Mesenteric ischaemia

Leg ulcers

- Venous ulcer
- Arterial ulcer
- Pyoderma gangrenosum
- Maligancy

Liver Cirrhosis

Viral hepatitis B, C

Alchohol

Primary biliary cirrhosis

Autoimmune hepatitis

Haemochromatosis

Wilson's disease

Drugs (eg. Methotrexate)

Non alcoholic steatohepatitis (NASH)

Alpha 1 antitrypsin deficiency

Secondary biliary cirrhosis

Congestive cardiac failure

Left Ventricular Failure

Ischaemic Heart Disease

Hypertension

Valvular heart disease
Mitral or Aortic

Cardiomyopathy

Volume Overload

Thyrotoxicosis

Septicaemia

Myocarditis

Infective endocarditis

Severe anaemia

Left Ventricular Failure (continued)

- Thiamine deficiency
- Arteriovenous Fistula
- Haemochromatosis
- Chaga's disease
- Drugs

Macrocytic anaemia

B12 deficiency

Folate deficiency

Haemolysis

Myelodysplastic Syndrome

Hypothroidism

Alcohol

Liver disease

Drugs

Malabsorbtion

Coeliac disease

Tropical sprue

Bacterial overgrowth

Giardiasis

Whipple's disease
(Tropheryma)

Intestinal infection

Drugs

Zollinger Ellison syndrome
(hypergastrinaemia)

Lymphoma

Intestinal lymphangiectasia

Malabsorbtion (continued)

Abetalipoproteinaemia

Protein losing enteropathy
    Crohn's disease

Tuberculosis (of gut)

Radiation enteritis

Bowel surgery

Pancreatic causes
    Chronic pancreatitis
    Carcinoma of the pancreas

Scleroderma

Amyloidosis

Mouth ulcers (Apthous)

Crohn's Disaese

Coeliac disease

Behcet's

Phemphigus

Phemphigoid

Syphilllis

Herpes simplex

Muscular dystrophies

- Duchenne
- Limb Girdle
- Myotonic
- Fascioscapulohumeral
- Oculopharyngeal

Myopathy

Congenital

Endocrine
- Diabetes
- Cushing's
- Thyrotoxicosis

Vitamin D deficiency

Drugs

Polymyositis

Nephrotic syndrome

Glomerulonephritis

Diabetes Mellitus

Amyloidosis

Systemic Lupus Erythematosus

Drugs

Malaria

Differential Diagnosis in General Medicine

Neurocutaneous syndromes

- Neurofibromatosis
- Tuberous sclerosis
- Von-hippel Lindau syndrome

Neutrophilia

- Bacterial infection
- Myeloproliferative disorder
- Steroids
- Haemorrhage
- Burns
- Polyarteritis nodosa
- Myocardial infarction

Normocytic anaemia

- Anaemia of chronic disease
- Renal failure
- Acute blood loss
- Haemolysis
- Hypothyroidism
- Mixed iron and B12/folate deficiency

Nystagmaus

Central

    Multiple Sclerosis
    Brain stem lesions
    Tumour
    Alcohol

Peripheral

    Labrynthitis
    Meniere's syndrome
    Acoustic neuroma

Obstructive Jaundice

Posthepatic
- Common bile duct stones
- Carcinoma of the head of the pancreas
- Cholangiocarcinoma
- Enlarged lymph nodes at porta hepatis
- Benign Stricture
- Primary sclerosing cholangitis

Intrahepatic
- Viral hepatitis
- Primary biliary cirrhosis
- Drugs (eg. Contraceptive Pill)
- Cholestasis of pregnancy

Optic atrophy

- Multiple sclerosis
- Tobacco
- Vitamin deficiency
- Pituitary mass

Differential Diagnosis in General Medicine

Pancytopenia

- Aplastic anaemia
- Myelodysplasia
- Myeloma
- Leukaemia
- Lymhoma
- Megaloblastic anaemia
- Drugs
- Hypersplenism

Papilloedema

Space occupying brain lesion

CO_2 retention

Hydrocephalus

Pericarditis

Viral
- Coxsackie
- Echo
- HIV

Bacterial
- Tuberculosis
- Pneumonia

Connective Tissue disorders
- Systemic Lupus Erythematosus
- Rheumatoid Arthritis

Post MI
- Acute MI
- Dressler's syndrome

Malignancy
- Primary
- Metastases

Pericarditis (continued)

- Ureamia
- Myxoedema
- Drugs
- Post-radiationm
- Post-surgical
- Postpericardiotomy syndrome

Peripheral Neuropathy

Diabetes

Non-metastatic manifestation of malignancy

Drugs (eg. Isoniazid)

Vitamin B12 deficiency

Alcohol

Guillam Barre syndrome

Connective tissue disease

Sarcoidosis

Amyloidosis

Hereditary sensory-motor neuropathy (eg. Charcot-Marie-Tooth)

Peripheral Neuropathy (continued)

Leprosy

HIV associated neuropathy

Peripheral nerve entrapment

Arteritis (eg. Polyarteritis nodosa)
Myeloma

Peroneal Nerve palsy

- Diabetes Mellitus
- Vascultiis
- Nerve compression
- Systemic Lupus Erythematosus
- Leprosy

Pleural effusion

Exudates

- Pneumonia
- Malignancy
- Tuberculosis
- Connective tissue disease eg. Systemic Lupus Erythematosus
- Pulmonary Embolism leading to pulmonary infarction
- Subphrenic abscess

Transudates

- Cardiac failure
- Hypoalbuminaemia (eg. Nephritic syndrome)

Differential Diagnosis in General Medicine

Polycythaemia

Polycythaemia Rubra Vera

Hypoxia – high altitude, cyanotic heart disease

Liver carcinoma

Renal carcinoma

Cerebellar haemangioma

Polyuria

- Diabetes Mellitus
- Diabetes insipidus (cranial, nephrogenic)
- Chronic renal failure
- Hypercalcaemia
- Hysterical polydypsia

Differential Diagnosis in General Medicine

Proteinuria

- Nephrotic syndrome
- Diabetes mellitus
- Hypertension
- Multiple myeloma

Proximal myopathy

- Diabetic amyotrophy
- Steroids
- Cushing's
- Polymyositis
- Thyrotoxicosis
- Carcinomatour neuropathy
- Muscular Dystrophy (Hereditary)

Purpura

Thrombocytopenia

Vasculitis
(including henoch-scholein purpura)

Steroids

Senile

Pyrexia of unknown origin

Abscess

Tuberculosis

Infective endocarditis

Human Immunodeficiency Virus (HIV)

Brucellosis

Lyme disease

Epstein-Barr Virus (EBV)

Cytomegalovirus (CMV)

Lymphoma

Renal cell carcinoma

Leukaemia

> **Pyrexia of unknown origin (continued)**

> Vasculitis
>
> Systemic Lupus Erythematosus
>
> Thyrotoxicosis
>
> Inflammatory Bowel Disease
>
> Sarcoidosis
>
> Drug fever
>
> Familial Mediterranean fever

Acute Coronary Syndrome

Family History

Hyperlipidaemia

Smoking

Diabetes

Hypertension

Heavy alcohol intake

Homocysteinaemia

Obesity

Splenomegaly

Infection
- Glandular fever (infectious mononucleosis)
- Typhoid
- Malaria
- Septicaemia
- Infective endocarditis
- Kala-Azar (Leishmaniasis)
- Tuberculosis
- Lyme disease (Borrelia infection)
- Weil's disease (leptospirosis)
- Brucellosis

Haematological
- Chronic myeloid leukaemia
- Haemolytic anaemia
- Myelofibrosis
- Primary polycythaemia

Splenomegaly (continued)

>
> Lymphoma
> Sickle cell anaemia
> Thalassaemia
> Pernicious anaemia
> Paraproteinaemia
>
> Portal Hypertension
> often due to liver cirrhosis
>
> Connective tissue disease
> Rheumatoid Arthritis
> Systemic Lupus Erythematosus
> Vasculitis
> Sjogren's syndrome
>
> Malignancy
>
> Others
> Sarcoidosis
> Gaucher's syndrome
> Amyloidosis

Seronegative arthritis

Ankolysing spondylitis

Psoriatic arthritis

Reactive arthritis

Reiter's disease

Enteropathic arthritis
(Inflammatory Bowel Disease)

Gout

Pseudogout
(pyrophosphate arthropathy)

Seronegative arthritis

Rheumatoid arthritis

Motor Neurone disease

Cervical Radiculopathy

Syringomyelia

Guillain barre Syndrome

Charco-marie-tooth

Bilateral cervical ribs

Pancoast syndrome: unilateral

Differential Diagnosis in General Medicine

Spastic paraparesis

Cord compression

Multiple sclerosis

Motor Neurone disease

Sub acute combined degeneration of the cord

Transverse myelitis

Syhillis

Cord infarction/arteritis

Para sagittal meningioma

Sagittal sinus thrombosis

Seronegative Arthritides

Ankylosing spondylitis

Enteropathic
(Inflammatory Bowel Disease)

Psoriatic arthritis

Reactive arthritis

Differential Diagnosis in General Medicine

Syncope

- Vasovagal attack
- Postural hypotension
- Drugs
- Heart block (second degree mobitz type two and third degree)
- Cardiac arrhythmias
- Aortic Stenosis
- Cough syncope
- Micturition syncope
- Carotid sunus syncope
- Effort syncope

Syncope (continued)

Pulmonary Embolism

Anaemia

Hypoglycaemia

Gastrointestinal bleed

Cyanotic congenital heart disease

Transient ischaemic attack

Vertebro-basilar insufficiency

Subclavian steal syndrome

Cardiomyopathy

Pacemaker failure

Tachycardia - Broad complex

Ventricular tachycardia

Supraventricular Tachycardia
(with aberrant conduction)

Tachycardia- Narrow complex

Supra Ventricular tachycardia

Atrial Fibrillation

Atrial flutter

Junctional tachycardia

Testicular pain

- Torsion
- Epididymo orchitis
- Inguinal hernia
- Hydrocele
- Varicocele
- Tumour

Thrombocytosis

- Haemorrhage
- Infection
- Malignancy
- Post –operative

Thrombophilia

Activated protein c resistance / Factor v leiden mutation

Protein c and protein S deficiency

Anti thrombin deficiency

Contraceptive pill

Tremor

- Parkinson's
- Cerebellar disease
- Thyrotoxicosis
- Alcoholism
- Benign essential tremor
- Drugs (salbutamol)
- Wilson's diasease

Uveitis

- Ankylosing spondylitis
- Sarcoidosis
- Inflammatory bowel disease
- Tuberculosis
- Behcet's syndrome
- Reiter's syndrome

Vasculitis

Polyarteritis Nodosa

Churg-strauss

Wegener's granulomatosis

Temporal arteritis

Drug induced

Henoch-schonlein purpura

Kawazaki disease

Takayashu's arteritis

Differential Diagnosis in General Medicine

Vomiting

- Gastroenteritis
- Cholecystitis
- Bowel Obstruction
- Viral infection
- Pyelonephritis
- Diabetic ketoacidosis
- Uraemia
- Pregnancy
- Alcohol
- Drugs
- Raised intracranial pressure

Vomiting (continued)

- Migraine
- Vestibular problems
- Hypercalcaemia

Differential Diagnosis in General Medicine

Wide splitting of heart sounds

Right Bundle Branch Block

Ventricular Septal Defect

Pulmonary stenosis

Mitral regurgitation

Atrial Septal Defect